SELF CARE

PLANNER

JOURNAL

♥

This Journal belongs to:

Getting Started

This Self-Care Planner & Journal prioritizes your wellness by default making it infinitely easier to create positive daily habits including sleep, exercise, diet, & more. With the help of The Self-Care Planner, you'll be able to achieve more without compromising your health and wellbeing in the process.
Our goal is to inspire you to take charge of your life, prioritize your time mindfully, and become the best version of yourself.

How to use it?

- Each Morning Go through the *Self-Care activities list* to get ideas for what you can do to take better care of yourself.

- Write down your daily self care *intentions* for your physical- mental- emotional and spiritual wellbeing

- At the end of the day complete the daily *Journal prompts*

- At the end of each week you'll have to complete a *Self Reflection Exercise that* will help you to better know yourself so that you can feel empowered and free

Look after yourself better and make Self Care an easy and regular part of your life with the help of this weekly Self-Care Planner, Journal and Workbook. Use this to check in with yourself regularly and improve your wellbeing, health and hapiness.

"Self-care is never a selfish act—it
is simply good stewardship of the
only gift I have, the gift I was put
on earth to offer to others."
Parker Palmer

♥

Self-care is vital for building resilience toward those
stressors in life that you can't eliminate. When you've
taken steps to care for your mind and body, you'll be
better equipped to live your best life.

♥

"It is so important to take time for
yourself and find clarity. The most
important relationship is the one you
have with yourself."
Diane Von Furstenberg

THE 7 PILLARS
of Self-Care

01
MENTAL
Mental self-care is about cultivating a healthy mindset through mindfulness and curiosity

02
EMOTIONAL
Emotional self-care involves taking care of your hear with healthy coping strategies.

03
PHYSICAL
Physical self-care involves taking care of your body with exercise, nutrition, and proper sleep.

04
ENVIRONMENTAL
Environmental self-care involves taking care of the spaces and places around you.

05
SPIRITUAL
Spiritual self-care involves activities or practices that give a sense of meaning to your life.

06
RECREATIONAL
Recreational self-care involves making time for hobbies, fun activities, and new experiences.

07
SOCIAL
Social self-care involves building relationships with regular connection and healthy boundaries.

Self Care Ideas

Here are some examples of what you can do to take better care of yourself in the various area of your life.

BODY

Go to the gym
Eat nourishing food
Drink more water
8 hours of sleep

MIND

Read more
Learn something new
Drawing
Watch a documentary

HEART

Talk with a friend
Be compassionate
Be present
Play/have fun
Rest/retreat

SOUL

Meditate
Light a candle
Journal
Time in nature
Give gratitude

Self Care Daily Planner

DATE:

AM ☀

S M T W T F S

What can I do today to take better care of myself?

Body

....

Mind

....

Heart

....

Soul

....

One Daily Positive Affirmation:

....

....

Self Care Daily Journal

DATE:

PM ☾

S M T W T F S

Things I did for myself today:

....

....

....

....

What is one thing you are proud about today?

....

....

I'm grateful for...

....

....

Self Care Daily Planner

DATE: _____   AM ☀

S M T W T F S

What can I do today to take better care of myself?

Body

....

Mind

....

Heart

....

Soul

....

One Daily Positive Affirmation:

....

....

Self Care Daily Journal

DATE:

PM ☾

S M T W T F S

Things I did for myself today:

....

....

....

....

What is one thing you are proud about today?

....

....

I'm grateful for...

....

....

Self Care Daily Planner

DATE:

AM ☼

S M T W T F S

What can I do today to take better care of myself?

Body

....

Mind

....

Heart

....

Soul

....

One Daily Positive Affirmation:

....

....

Self Care Daily Journal

DATE:

PM 🌙

S M T W T F S

Things I did for myself today:

....

....

....

....

What is one thing you are proud about today?

....

....

I'm grateful for...

....

....

Self Care Daily Planner

DATE:

AM ☀

S M T W T F S

What can I do today to take better care of myself?

Body

....

Mind

....

Heart

....

Soul

....

One Daily Positive Affirmation:

....

....

Self Care Daily Journal

DATE: PM ☾

S M T W T F S

Things I did for myself today:

....

....

....

....

What is one thing you are proud about today?

....

....

I'm grateful for...

....

....

Self Care Daily Planner

DATE: AM ☀

S M T W T F S

What can I do today to take better care of myself?

Body

....

Mind

....

Heart

....

Soul

....

One Daily Positive Affirmation:

....

....

Self Care Daily Journal

DATE: PM ☾

S M T W T F S

Things I did for myself today:

....

....

....

....

What is one thing you are proud about today?

....

....

I'm grateful for...

....

....

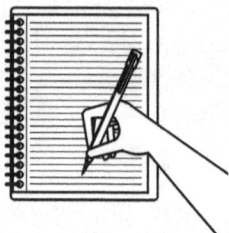

Weekly Self-Reflection Exercise

Reflection and Realization

A journal allows you to freely express yourself without fear of disapproval or criticism. Not only is it a good outlet, but it is also a way to sharpen your writing skills.

On this page, write about a significant event that shifted your perspective.

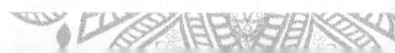

self-care check-in

EAT THREE MAIN MEALS

GO ON A 24-HOUR SOCIAL MEDIA DETOX

FIND A QUIET SPOT TO MEDITATE

LIGHT AN AROMATIC CANDLE

DO A GRATITUDE LIST

PRACTICE DEEP BREATHING

LISTEN TO GOOD MUSIC

EXERCISE

CATCH UP WITH A FRIEND

VISIT A FAMILY MEMBER

SPEND TIME OUTDOORS

HAVE A MINI PAMPER SESH

CUDDLE A PET

TRY SOMETHING NEW

READ A BOOK

Make it a habit to take care of yourself

Self Care Daily Planner

DATE:

AM ☀

S M T W T F S

What can I do today to take better care of myself?

Body

....

Mind

....

Heart

....

Soul

....

One Daily Positive Affirmation:

....

....

Self Care Daily Journal

DATE:

PM 🌙

S M T W T F S

Things I did for myself today:

....

....

....

....

What is one thing you are proud about today?

....

....

I'm grateful for...

....

....

Self Care Daily Planner

DATE:

AM ☀

S M T W T F S

What can I do today to take better care of myself?

Body

....

Mind

....

Heart

....

Soul

....

One Daily Positive Affirmation:

....

....

Self Care Daily Journal

DATE: PM ☽

S M T W T F S

Things I did for myself today:

....

....

....

....

What is one thing you are proud about today?

....

....

I'm grateful for...

....

....

Self Care Daily Planner

DATE:

AM ☀

S M T W T F S

What can I do today to take better care of myself?

Body

....

Mind

....

Heart

....

Soul

....

One Daily Positive Affirmation:

....

....

Self Care Daily Journal

DATE:

PM ☾

S M T W T F S

Things I did for myself today:

....

....

....

....

What is one thing you are proud about today?

....

....

I'm grateful for...

....

....

Self Care Daily Planner

DATE:

AM ☼

S M T W T F S

What can I do today to take better care of myself?

Body

....

Mind

....

Heart

....

Soul

....

One Daily Positive Affirmation:

....

....

Self Care Daily Journal

DATE:

PM ☾

S M T W T F S

Things I did for myself today:

....

....

....

....

What is one thing you are proud about today?

....

....

I'm grateful for...

....

....

Self Care Daily Planner

DATE:

AM ☀

S M T W T F S

What can I do today to take better care of myself?

Body

....

Mind

....

Heart

....

Soul

....

One Daily Positive Affirmation:

....

....

Self Care Daily Journal

DATE:

PM ☽

S M T W T F S

Things I did for myself today:

....

....

....

....

What is one thing you are proud about today?

....

....

I'm grateful for...

....

....

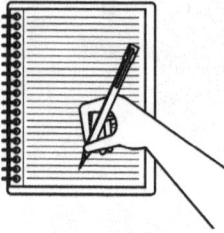

Weekly Self-Reflection Exercise

Strengths and Weaknesses

Make a list of three qualities you have that you consider weaknesses, then explore how these so-called weaknesses might be recast as strengths. For instance, if you believe micromanagement is a weakness of yours, it could also mean that you're organised and responsible. Once you determine the strength on the flip side of that quality, write about a time when you used that quality in a positive way.

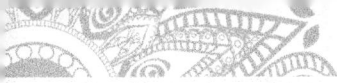

Self-Reflection - Strengths and Weaknesses

Self-Care Ideas for this Week

Get up and dance.

Enjoy a good meal.

Take three deep breaths.

Go offline for a day.

Sing your favorite song.

Meditate for a few minutes.

Take a nap.

Remember a good memory.

Plan next week's menu.

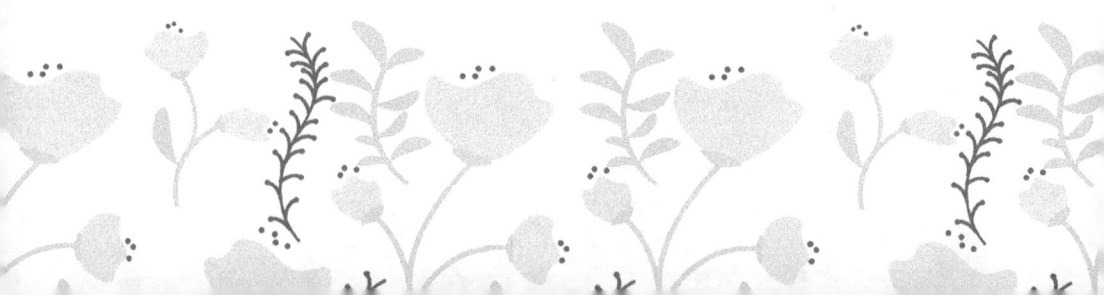

Say Nice Things To Yourself!

"I look good wearing shorts!"

"I like my new haircut!"

"Wow, my face is really bright today!"

"New day, new stuff to learn!"

"Myself is my top priority!"

"I look gorgeous!"

"I would like to date myself"

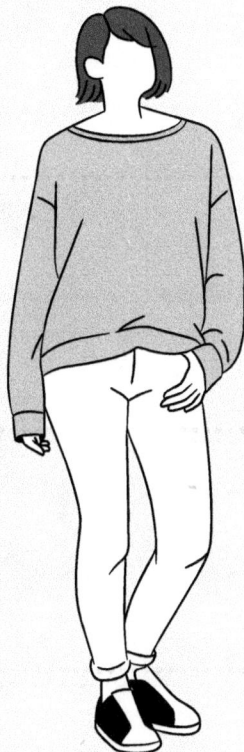

Don't be shy to say nice things to yourself, accept those compliments because you deserve it!

Self Care Daily Planner

DATE:

AM ☀

S M T W T F S

What can I do today to take better care of myself?

Body

....

Mind

....

Heart

....

Soul

....

One Daily Positive Affirmation:

....

....

Self Care Daily Journal

DATE: PM ☾

S M T W T F S

Things I did for myself today:

....

....

....

....

What is one thing you are proud about today?

....

....

I'm grateful for...

....

....

Self Care Daily Planner

DATE:

AM ☀

S M T W T F S

What can I do today to take better care of myself?

Body

....

Mind

....

Heart

....

Soul

....

One Daily Positive Affirmation:

....

....

Self Care Daily Journal

DATE:

PM ☾

S M T W T F S

Things I did for myself today:

....

....

....

....

What is one thing you are proud about today?

....

....

I'm grateful for...

....

....

Self Care Daily Planner

DATE:

AM ☀

S M T W T F S

What can I do today to take better care of myself?

Body

....

Mind

....

Heart

....

Soul

....

One Daily Positive Affirmation:

....

....

Self Care Daily Journal

DATE:

PM ☾

S M T W T F S

Things I did for myself today:

....

....

....

....

What is one thing you are proud about today?

....

....

I'm grateful for...

....

....

Self Care Daily Planner

DATE:

AM ☀

S M T W T F S

What can I do today to take better care of myself?

Body

....

Mind

....

Heart

....

Soul

....

One Daily Positive Affirmation:

....

....

Self Care Daily Journal

DATE:

PM ☾

S M T W T F S

Things I did for myself today:

....

....

....

....

What is one thing you are proud about today?

....

....

I'm grateful for...

....

....

Self Care Daily Planner

DATE:

AM ☀

S M T W T F S

What can I do today to take better care of myself?

Body

....

Mind

....

Heart

....

Soul

....

One Daily Positive Affirmation:

....

....

Self Care Daily Journal

DATE: PM ☾

S M T W T F S

Things I did for myself today:

....

....

....

....

What is one thing you are proud about today?

....

....

I'm grateful for...

....

....

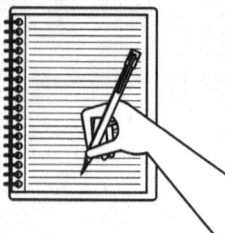

Weekly Self-Reflection Exercise

Define your Intentions

List five qualities of your personality or your outlook that you think defines you. Write just one word/ phrase/sentence for each—not a summary of your whole life. Don't overthink. What rises to the surface as important now? You can even do this prompt periodically to see how the list changes. Then expand on the qualities, writing about each of those aspects of you..

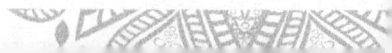

Self-Care Bingo

TAKE A SHOWER	GET DRESSED	GET IN TOUCH WITH FRIENDS	PROCESS MY FEELINGS	COMPLIMENT MYSELF
MEDITATE	EAT GOOD FOOD	LISTEN TO MY BODY	HAVE FUN	ASK FOR HELP
TAKE A MUCH - NEEDED BREAK	DRINK WATER	*Free*	TAKE A SOCIAL MEDIA BREAK	TREAT MYSELF
COMPLIMENT SOMEONE	GET 8 HOURS OF SLEEP	TAKE STEPS TO TAME NEGATIVE THOUGHTS	HUG MY PARENTS	BREAK A HABIT THAT IS NOT FOR ME
TAKE A MENTAL HEALTH DAY	SPEND TIME IN NATURE	DECLUTTER MY SPACE	WRITE DOWN IN MY JOURNAL	PRACTICE SELF - COMPASSION

Self Care Daily Planner

DATE:

AM ☼

S M T W T F S

What can I do today to take better care of myself?

Body

....

Mind

....

Heart

....

Soul

....

One Daily Positive Affirmation:

....

....

Self Care Daily Journal

DATE:

PM 🌙

S M T W T F S

Things I did for myself today:

....

....

....

....

What is one thing you are proud about today?

....

....

I'm grateful for...

....

....

Self Care Daily Planner

DATE:

AM ☀

S M T W T F S

What can I do today to take better care of myself?

Body

....

Mind

....

Heart

....

Soul

....

One Daily Positive Affirmation:

....

....

Self Care Daily Journal

DATE:

PM 🌙

S M T W T F S

Things I did for myself today:

....

....

....

....

What is one thing you are proud about today?

....

....

I'm grateful for...

....

....

Self Care Daily Planner

DATE: AM ☼

S M T W T F S

What can I do today to take better care of myself?

Body

....

Mind

....

Heart

....

Soul

....

One Daily Positive Affirmation:

....

....

Self Care Daily Journal

DATE:

PM 🌙

S M T W T F S

Things I did for myself today:

....

....

....

....

What is one thing you are proud about today?

....

....

I'm grateful for...

....

....

Self Care Daily Planner

DATE:

AM ☀

S M T W T F S

What can I do today to take better care of myself?

Body

....

Mind

....

Heart

....

Soul

....

One Daily Positive Affirmation:

....

....

Self Care Daily Journal

DATE:

PM 🌙

S M T W T F S

Things I did for myself today:

....

....

....

....

What is one thing you are proud about today?

....

....

I'm grateful for...

....

....

Self Care Daily Planner

DATE:

AM ☀

S M T W T F S

What can I do today to take better care of myself?

Body

....

Mind

....

Heart

....

Soul

....

One Daily Positive Affirmation:

....

....

Self Care Daily Journal

DATE:

PM 🌙

S M T W T F S

Things I did for myself today:

....

....

....

....

What is one thing you are proud about today?

....

....

I'm grateful for...

....

....

DATE _____

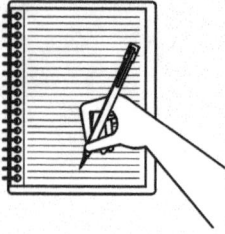

Weekly Self-Reflection Exercise

Make Time for Joy

List three activities that bring you joy. Expand on each activity, describing a recent time when you fully engaged in it. If you're finding it challenging to engage in these activities as often as you'd like or need, explore strategies for working them into your schedule more often.

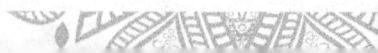

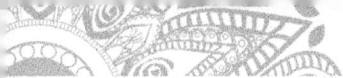

Self-Reflection - Make Time for Joy

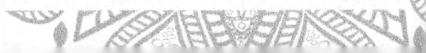

SELF-CARE
CHECK OUT

What you could do this Week

••

Going out for a stroll	$0.00
Simple stretching	$0.00
Eating favorite salad	$0.00
Watching favorite show	$0.00
Listen to music	$0.00
Use mud mask	$0.00
Text friends	$0.00
Greet neighbours	$0.00
Have a cat nap	$0.00
Buy yourself flowers	$0.00
Dance like crazy	$0.00
Try Yoga	$0.00

••

Total: **$0.00**

0000000000000000

Because simple things require no money

Self Care Daily Planner

DATE:

AM ☼

S M T W T F S

What can I do today to take better care of myself?

Body

....

Mind

....

Heart

....

Soul

....

One Daily Positive Affirmation:

....

....

Self Care Daily Journal

Things I did for myself today:

....

....

....

....

What is one thing you are proud about today?

....

....

I'm grateful for...

....

....

Self Care Daily Planner

DATE:

AM ☼

S M T W T F S

What can I do today to take better care of myself?

Body

....

Mind

....

Heart

....

Soul

....

One Daily Positive Affirmation:

....

....

Self Care Daily Journal

DATE:

PM ☾

S M T W T F S

Things I did for myself today:

....

....

....

....

What is one thing you are proud about today?

....

....

I'm grateful for...

....

....

Self Care Daily Planner

DATE:

AM ☼

S M T W T F S

What can I do today to take better care of myself?

Body

....

Mind

....

Heart

....

Soul

....

One Daily Positive Affirmation:

....

....

Self Care Daily Journal

DATE: PM ☾

S M T W T F S

Things I did for myself today:

....

....

....

....

What is one thing you are proud about today?

....

....

I'm grateful for...

....

....

Self Care Daily Planner

DATE:

AM ☼

S M T W T F S

What can I do today to take better care of myself?

Body

....

Mind

....

Heart

....

Soul

....

One Daily Positive Affirmation:

....

....

Self Care Daily Journal

DATE: PM 🌙

S M T W T F S

Things I did for myself today:

....

....

....

....

What is one thing you are proud about today?

....

....

I'm grateful for...

....

....

Self Care Daily Planner

DATE:

AM ☀

S M T W T F S

What can I do today to take better care of myself?

Body

....

Mind

....

Heart

....

Soul

....

One Daily Positive Affirmation:

....

....

Self Care Daily Journal

DATE: PM ☾

S M T W T F S

Things I did for myself today:

....

....

....

....

What is one thing you are proud about today?

....

....

I'm grateful for...

....

....

DATE _____

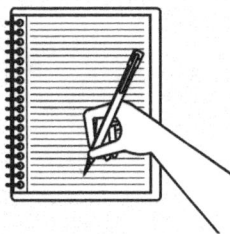

Weekly Self-Reflection Exercise

Discover your Self Place

Think of a real or an imaginary place where you feel safe and at peace. Create that place in your mind and write a detailed description of it using all your senses—what you see in this place, but also what you hear, smell, taste, and feel through tactile contact. You can then use this as a visualized meditation, closing your eyes, breathing, and imagining this place thoroughly, one sense at a time.

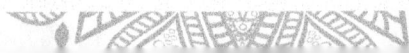

Self-Reflection - Discover your Safe Place

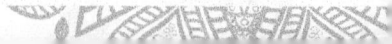

20 Self-Care Ideas to Help You Through a Bad Day

- ♥ SPENT TIME WITH PEOPLE WHO LIFT YOU UP
- ♥ GET YOUR HAIR DONE
- ♥ SLEEP IN OR TAKE A NAP
- ♥ SCHEDULE IN SOME ME-TIME DOING SOMETHING YOU ENJOY
- ♥ CALL A FRIEND
- ♥ WATCH YOUR FAVOURITE SHOW OR MOVIE
- ♥ HEAD OUTSIDE FOR A WALK IN THE FRESH AIR
- ♥ SINK YOUR TEETH INTO A GOOD BOOK
- ♥ EXERCISE
- ♥ TAKE A MENTAL HEALTHY DAY
- ♥ NOURISH YOUR BODY BY EATING AND DRINKING HEALTHY FOR THE DAY
- ♥ SPEND TIME WITH ANIMALS
- ♥ MEDITATE
- ♥ SPEND TIME WITH SOMEONE UNDER THE AGE OF 6 OR OVER THE AGE OF 60
- ♥ HIT THE SHOPS FOR SOME RETAIL THERAPY
- ♥ LUXURIATE IN A LONG, HOT SHOWE OR BATH
- ♥ WRITE YOUR THOUGHTS OUT IN YOUR JOURNAL
- ♥ DECLARE A COUCH DAY
- ♥ SPEND TIME IN NATURE
- ♥ UNPLUG

Self Care Daily Planner

DATE:

AM ☀

S M T W T F S

What can I do today to take better care of myself?

Body

....

Mind

....

Heart

....

Soul

....

One Daily Positive Affirmation:

....

....

Self Care Daily Journal

DATE:

PM 🌙

S M T W T F S

Things I did for myself today:

....

....

....

....

What is one thing you are proud about today?

....

....

I'm grateful for...

....

....

Self Care Daily Planner

DATE:

AM ☀

S M T W T F S

What can I do today to take better care of myself?

Body

....

Mind

....

Heart

....

Soul

....

One Daily Positive Affirmation:

....

....

Self Care Daily Journal

DATE:

PM ☾

S M T W T F S

Things I did for myself today:

....

....

....

....

What is one thing you are proud about today?

....

....

I'm grateful for...

....

....

Self Care Daily Planner

DATE:

AM ☀

S M T W T F S

What can I do today to take better care of myself?

Body

....

Mind

....

Heart

....

Soul

....

One Daily Positive Affirmation:

....

....

Self Care Daily Journal

DATE: PM ☾

S M T W T F S

Things I did for myself today:

··

··

··

··

What is one thing you are proud about today?

··

··

I'm grateful for...

··

··

Self Care Daily Planner

DATE:

AM ☀

S M T W T F S

What can I do today to take better care of myself?

Body

....

Mind

....

Heart

....

Soul

....

One Daily Positive Affirmation:

....

....

Self Care Daily Journal

DATE:

PM ☾

S M T W T F S

Things I did for myself today:

....

....

....

....

What is one thing you are proud about today?

....

....

I'm grateful for...

....

....

Self Care Daily Planner

DATE:

AM ☀

S M T W T F S

What can I do today to take better care of myself?

Body

....

Mind

....

Heart

....

Soul

....

One Daily Positive Affirmation:

....

....

Self Care Daily Journal

DATE:

PM ☾

S M T W T F S

Things I did for myself today:

....

....

....

....

What is one thing you are proud about today?

....

....

I'm grateful for...

....

....

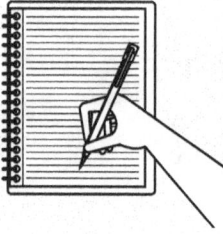

Weekly Self-Reflection Exercise

Create a Balance

LList two things you tend to say yes to or have said yes to recently and two things you tend to say no to or have said no to recently. What was good self-care and what wasn't? For example, saying yes can be a way of embracing an opportunity and engaging with the world (good self-care), but it can also be a way of spreading yourself too thin. Saying no can help you maintain healthy boundaries and manage your time (good self-care), but it can also isolate you and cause you to miss opportunities. This awareness can help you prioritize, and determine the value of things and what's truly important to you

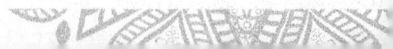

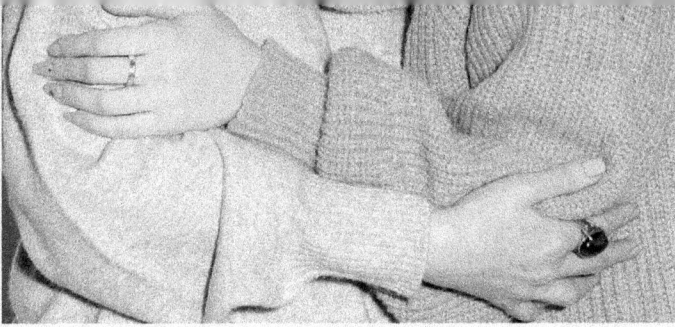

Self Love Bingo

Your Daily Check of Self Love

Say "I'm Beautiful" In Front of The Mirror	Take A Bath	Listen to Your Favorite Music
Use Face Mask	Take An Afternoon Nap	Eat Your Favorite Snack
Try Different Style of Clothes	Doodle Anything On A Paper	Gaze At The Afternoon Sky

You Should Self-Love Today Too

I Tag My Loveliest Friend :

_____

Self - Esteem Bingo

MASTER A NEW SKILL	LET NEGATIVE PEOPLE GO	STAND AT THE EDGE OF COMFORT ZONE	DO SOMETHING CREATIVE OFTEN	AFFIRM YOURSELF OFTEN
EXPRESS FEELINGS	ACCEPT FAILURES AS PART OF GROWTH	FACE FEARS	MANAGE TIME WELL	MAKE TIME FOR REST
EXERCISE OFTEN	CULTIVATE HOBBIES	*Free*	LIVE HUMBLY	BE KIND TO YOURSELF
HONOR YOUR WORD TO OTHERS	REMIND YOURSELF YOU ARE ENOUGH	LOVE YOURSELF MORE THAN OTHERS WILL	DREAM BIG AND MAKE IT HAPPEN	CHALLENGE LIMITING BELIEFS
HELP SOMEONE	STOP WORRYING ABOUT WHAT OTHERS THINK	HEAL YOUR PAST	READ SOMETHING INSPIRATIONAL	RECLAIM INTEGRITY

Self Care Daily Planner

DATE:

AM ☀

S M T W T F S

What can I do today to take better care of myself?

Body

....

Mind

....

Heart

....

Soul

....

One Daily Positive Affirmation:

....

....

Self Care Daily Journal

Things I did for myself today:

....

....

....

....

What is one thing you are proud about today?

....

....

I'm grateful for...

....

....

Self Care Daily Planner

DATE:

AM ☀

S M T W T F S

What can I do today to take better care of myself?

Body

....

Mind

....

Heart

....

Soul

....

One Daily Positive Affirmation:

....

....

Self Care Daily Journal

DATE:

PM ☾

S M T W T F S

Things I did for myself today:

....

....

....

....

What is one thing you are proud about today?

....

....

I'm grateful for...

....

....

Self Care Daily Planner

DATE:

AM ☀

S M T W T F S

What can I do today to take better care of myself?

Body

....

Mind

....

Heart

....

Soul

....

One Daily Positive Affirmation:

....

....

Self Care Daily Journal

DATE: PM ☾

S M T W T F S

Things I did for myself today:

....

....

....

....

What is one thing you are proud about today?

....

....

I'm grateful for...

....

....

Self Care Daily Planner

DATE:

AM ☀

S M T W T F S

What can I do today to take better care of myself?

Body

....

Mind

....

Heart

....

Soul

....

One Daily Positive Affirmation:

....

....

Self Care Daily Journal

DATE:

PM ☾

S M T W T F S

Things I did for myself today:

....

....

....

....

What is one thing you are proud about today?

....

....

I'm grateful for...

....

....

Self Care Daily Planner

DATE:

AM ☼

S M T W T F S

What can I do today to take better care of myself?

Body

....

Mind

....

Heart

....

Soul

....

One Daily Positive Affirmation:

....

....

Self Care Daily Journal

DATE: PM ☾

S M T W T F S

Things I did for myself today:

....

....

....

....

What is one thing you are proud about today?

....

....

I'm grateful for...

....

....

DATE _____

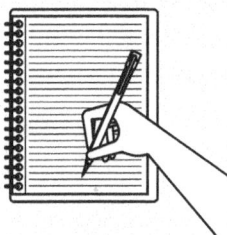

Weekly Self-Reflection Exercise

Develop Self Compassion

Journaling is an effective way to express emotions, and has been found to enhance both mental and physical well-being. Write down anything that you felt bad about, anything you judged yourself for, or any difficult experience that caused you pain. For each event, use mindfulness, a sense of common humanity, and kindness to process the event in a more self-compassionate way.Write yourself some kind, understanding, words of comfort. Let yourself know that you care about yourself, adopting a gentle, reassuring tone.

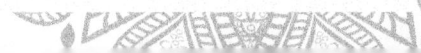

Self-Reflection - Dievelop Self Compassion

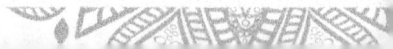

Want free goodies?

Thank You

so much for trying our Self-Care Planner!
We'd love to hear from you!

If you've found this to be a good book please,
support us and leave a review.

If you have any suggestions or issues with this book, or if
you want to test some of our latest notebooks
please email us.

Send email to:

pickme.readme@**gmail.com**

www.ingramcontent.com/pod-product-compliance
Lightning Source LLC
Chambersburg PA
CBHW070027030426
42335CB00017B/2324